Stress-Less

A Modern Guide to Mastering Your Mental Health in the 21st Century

By

Maynard Mene

Table of Content

Acknowledgement

I would like to extend my heartfelt thanks to all those who played a role in the creation and publication of my book, "Stress-Less: A Modern Guide to Mastering Your Mental Health in the 21st Century".

First and foremost, I am grateful to a higher power for providing me with the strength and guidance to bring this project to fruition.

I would also like to express my sincere gratitude to my wife, Edith, who was a pillar of support and encouragement throughout this journey. Her love and belief in me provided me with the motivation to keep going.

To my children, Oritsenela, Seuntola, and Molagbemi, I cannot thank you enough for your understanding and patience during this process. Your unwavering support and love have been a source of inspiration and pride for me.

Finally, I would like to acknowledge all the individuals who helped bring this book to life. Your contributions, support, and belief in this project have been invaluable, and I am grateful for your involvement.

Introduction.

1.1 Definition of Stress

Stress is a complex and multifaceted phenomenon that touches the essence of our being, both physically and psychologically. It is a natural response of our bodies to challenges, perceived threats, and difficult situations that we encounter in our daily lives. Though it can have both positive and negative effects, stress is a force that can be harnessed and managed with the right tools and knowledge.

Stress is defined as the dynamic interplay between the mind and the body in response to a perceived challenge or threat. This challenge can come from various sources, including external stressors such as a demanding work project, a troubled relationship, or a health concern. Additionally, stress can stem from internal stressors, such as self-doubt, anxiety, and worry.

When faced with a stressor, our bodies activate the "fight or flight" response, a primordial survival mechanism that prepares our bodies to respond to danger. Our brains release stress hormones such as cortisol and adrenaline, which increase heart rate, blood pressure, and blood sugar levels. This response is intended to provide energy and strength to our bodies, enabling us to tackle the perceived threat.

However, when stress becomes chronic and prolonged, it can have devastating consequences on our minds and bodies. Chronic stress can contribute to a host of health problems, including anxiety, depression, heart disease, and other illnesses. It can also affect our sleep, memory, and concentration, leading to feelings of exhaustion, irritability, and overwhelm.

Stress is a normal response to challenging situations, but when it becomes chronic, it can have negative effects on the mind and body. Understanding the definition of stress and the impact it can have on our lives is the first step in learning to manage stress and achieving a more balanced, stress-free life. With the right knowledge and tools, we can turn stress from a hindrance into a catalyst for growth, self-discovery, and resilience.

Chapter 1: Understanding Stress

Stress is a common experience in modern life, affecting people of all ages, backgrounds, and professions. Despite its prevalence, however, stress remains a poorly understood and often undervalued phenomenon. In this chapter, we will delve deeper into the nature of stress and what it means to our lives.

Definition of Stress - Stress is defined as the psychological and physiological response to a perceived challenge or threat. This challenge can come from external sources, such as work, relationships, or health concerns, or from internal sources, such as self-doubt, anxiety, or worry. When faced with a stressor, the body activates its "fight or flight" response, preparing the body to respond to danger.

The Positive and Negative Effects of Stress - While stress can have both positive and negative effects, it is important to understand that chronic stress can have serious consequences for our mental and physical health. Prolonged stress can lead to anxiety, depression, heart disease, and other illnesses, as well as affect sleep, memory, and concentration.

The Origin of Stress - The "fight or flight" response is a primitive survival mechanism that has evolved over millions of years to protect the body from danger. However, in the modern world, we are faced with a different type of stressor, one that is often less tangible and less immediate than the threats our ancestors faced. This new type of stressor requires a different approach to stress management.

1. The Impact of Modern Life - The fast-paced, high-pressure nature of modern life, combined with the constant exposure to news and social media, has increased the level of stress many people experience. It is important to understand how these factors contribute to stress and the impact they can have on our lives.

2.1 Physical and Psychological Effects of Stress

Stress is a complex phenomenon that affects both the mind and body in ways that can be far-reaching and long-lasting. When faced with a stressor, the body activates its "fight or flight" response, which prepares it to respond to danger. This response is intended to provide energy and strength to the body, but when it becomes prolonged and chronic, it can have negative effects on our physical and mental health.

1 Physical Effects of Stress - Chronic stress can contribute to a range of physical health problems, including heart disease, high blood pressure, digestive issues, headaches, and a weakened immune system. These physical effects of stress can make it difficult to carry out daily activities, and can also have long-term consequences for our overall health.

2 Psychological Effects of Stress - Prolonged stress can also take a toll on our mental health, contributing to anxiety, depression, irritability, and feelings of overwhelm. It can also negatively impact sleep, memory, and concentration, making it difficult to perform even simple tasks. The psychological effects of stress can be particularly challenging to manage, as they are often intertwined with our thoughts and emotions.

Therefore, understanding the physical and psychological effects of stress is critical in developing strategies to effectively manage it. By recognizing the impact that stress can have on our health and well-being, we can take steps to reduce its negative effects and maintain a more balanced, stress-free life. Whether you are just starting to grapple with stress or have been managing it for years, understanding the effects of stress is the first step in developing a plan for reducing its impact on your life.

2.2 Common Stress Triggers in the 21st Century

Stress is a ubiquitous part of modern life, and it can come from a variety of sources. In the 21st century, the pace of life has accelerated, and the demands of work and personal life can be overwhelming. As a result, it's no surprise that stress is one of the most common health problems facing people today.

1 Work-Related Stress - In today's fast-paced work environment, job stress is a major source of stress for many people. Long hours, demanding deadlines, and the pressure to perform at a high level can take a toll on our mental and physical health. Additionally, job insecurity and a lack of control over our work environment can also contribute to stress.

2 Technology Stress - The rise of technology has revolutionized the way we live, but it has also created new sources of stress. From the constant need to be connected to our devices, to the barrage of information that bombards us on a daily basis, technology stress is becoming an increasingly common trigger for stress in the 21st century.

3 Financial Stress - Money is a major source of stress for many people, and it can be particularly challenging in the 21st century where the cost of living is rising faster than salaries. The fear of losing a job, being unable to pay bills, or not having enough savings for retirement can all contribute to financial stress.

4 Relationship Stress - Relationships are a source of joy and fulfillment, but they can also be a source of stress. Whether it's navigating conflict with a partner, dealing with difficult family dynamics, or simply trying to find time for the people we care about, relationship stress can be a major trigger for stress in the 21st century.

2.3 Identifying Personal Stressors

Stress affects everyone differently, and the triggers that cause stress can vary greatly from person to person. While common stress triggers, such as work and relationships, can have a significant impact on our lives, it's equally important to understand the unique stressors that are specific to our own lives.

1 Personal Reflection - To identify personal stressors, it's helpful to start by reflecting on your own life and experiences. What causes you to feel stressed? What are the situations or circumstances that trigger stress for you? By taking the time to reflect on your own experiences, you can gain a deeper understanding of what causes stress in your life.

2 Keeping a Stress Journal - Keeping a stress journal can be a helpful tool in identifying personal stressors. Writing down what causes you to feel stressed, and how you respond to stress, can help you see patterns and trends in your behavior. This information can be valuable in developing strategies for managing stress.

3 Seeking Professional Help - If you are struggling to identify your personal stressors, or if you are experiencing stress that is affecting your quality of life, it may be helpful to seek professional help. A mental health professional can help you understand the underlying causes of stress and develop strategies for managing it.

Chapter 2: Mindfulness and Relaxation Techniques

3.1 Benefits of Mindfulness

Mindfulness is a simple yet powerful tool for reducing stress and improving well-being. By focusing on the present moment and accepting our thoughts and feelings without judgment, mindfulness can help us cultivate inner peace, reduce anxiety, and improve our overall sense of well-being.

1 Reduced Stress - One of the most significant benefits of mindfulness is its ability to reduce stress. By focusing on the present moment, mindfulness helps us to let go of worries and concerns, allowing us to relax and release built-up tension. This reduction in stress can lead to a range of positive effects, including improved sleep, enhanced memory and concentration, and a greater sense of happiness and well-being.

2 Improved Mental Health - Mindfulness has also been shown to have a positive impact on mental health. By helping us to understand and manage our thoughts and emotions, mindfulness can reduce symptoms of anxiety and depression, and improve our overall mood and well-being.

3 Increased Resilience - Mindfulness can also help us become more resilient, allowing us to better manage stress and other challenges in our lives. By cultivating inner peace and acceptance, mindfulness can help us develop a more positive outlook, enabling us to approach life with greater clarity, confidence, and peace of mind.

3.2 Mindfulness Exercises and Techniques

Mindfulness is a state of active and non-judgemental awareness of the present moment. It can be cultivated through a variety of mindfulness exercises and techniques that help us focus our attention on the present moment and develop a more mindful and relaxed state of mind.

1 Meditation - Meditation is one of the most popular and well-known mindfulness exercises. It involves sitting quietly and focusing on your breath, your body, or a specific object. By practising meditation regularly, you can develop greater mindfulness, reduce stress, and improve your mental and emotional well-being.

2 Body Scanning - Body scanning is a mindfulness exercise that involves lying down and focusing your attention on each part of your body, from your toes to the top of your head. By focusing on the sensations in each part of your body, you can release tension, reduce stress, and increase relaxation.

3 Mindful Breathing - Mindful breathing is a simple yet powerful mindfulness exercise that involves focusing on your breath and counting each inhale and exhale. By focusing on your breath, you can calm your mind and reduce stress, helping you to feel more relaxed and centered.

4 Mindful Walking - Mindful walking is a form of mindfulness that involves walking slowly and mindfully, focusing on your sensations, breath, and surroundings. By practising mindful walking, you can bring a sense of calm and relaxation to your daily life and reduce stress.

5 Yoga and Tai Chi - Yoga and Tai Chi are ancient practices that involve moving the body mindfully and in harmony with the breath. By practicing yoga or Tai Chi regularly, you can improve your flexibility, balance, and relaxation, and reduce stress and anxiety.

These mindfulness exercises and techniques can be incorporated into your daily routine and adapted to fit your individual needs and preferences. By practicing mindfulness regularly, you can increase your awareness of the present moment, reduce stress, and improve your overall well-being.

3.3 Relaxation Techniques for Stress Management

Relaxation techniques have been proven to be effective in reducing stress, promoting relaxation, and improving overall well-being. By intentionally slowing down and calming the mind and body, we can counteract the physical and psychological effects of stress and enhance our overall health and happiness.

There are many different types of relaxation techniques, each with its own set of benefits. Some popular techniques include:

Deep breathing: This technique involves focusing on breathing deeply and slowly, and allowing the body to relax. This can be done in any position and can be practiced for a few minutes a day to reduce stress and promote calm.

Progressive muscle relaxation: This technique involves tensing and then relaxing different muscle groups, starting with the feet and moving up the body. This helps to release tension in the muscles and reduce stress.

Guided imagery: This technique involves imagining a peaceful, calming scene, such as a beach or a forest, in order to bring a sense of calm and relaxation to the mind and body.

Yoga: This practice combines physical postures, controlled breathing, and meditation to promote relaxation and reduce stress.

Tai chi: This gentle form of exercise is characterized by slow, fluid movements and deep breathing, making it an excellent way to reduce stress and improve relaxation.

Meditation: This practice involves sitting quietly and focusing on the present moment, letting go of thoughts and worries. Meditation has been shown to reduce stress and promote relaxation, as well as improve mood, sleep, and overall health.

It is important to find the relaxation technique that works best for you and make it a part of your daily routine. Experiment with different techniques, and remember that the most important thing is to find a technique that you enjoy and can stick with long-term.

By incorporating relaxation techniques into your daily routine, you can effectively manage stress and improve your overall well-being. Whether you're looking to reduce stress, improve sleep, or simply bring more peace and calm into your life, these techniques can help you achieve your goals and live a more balanced, stress-free life.

Chapter 3: Healthy Habits for Stress Management

4.1 The Importance of Sleep for Stress Management

As the 21st century continues to bring a fast-paced and demanding lifestyle, it is more important than ever to prioritize self-care and adopt healthy habits for stress management. One of the most crucial components of stress management is ensuring adequate and quality sleep.

Sleep is essential for physical and mental well-being, and it plays a crucial role in managing stress levels. When we sleep, our bodies go through a series of physiological processes that help to repair and rejuvenate the body and mind. Adequate sleep helps to reduce stress hormones and increase the production of neurotransmitters that are essential for good mental health.

Chronic sleep deprivation is a common problem in the modern world, and it can have a significant impact on overall health and well-being. Lack of sleep can exacerbate stress levels and contribute to a range of physical and mental health problems, including depression, anxiety, heart disease, and obesity.

On the other hand, getting enough quality sleep can help to lower stress levels, improve mood, boost mental clarity, and enhance physical performance. A good night's sleep can help to improve memory, boost immunity, and increase resilience to stress.

4.2 Eating for Stress Management

Eating habits play a crucial role in stress management. When we're stressed, it's easy to fall into unhealthy patterns such as overeating junk food or skipping meals. However, these habits can actually increase stress levels and harm our physical and mental well-being. On the other hand, maintaining a balanced and nutritious diet can help reduce stress and improve overall health.

Eating a variety of nutrient-rich foods, including whole grains, fruits, vegetables, lean protein, and healthy fats, can help provide the body with the energy and nutrients it needs to cope with stress. Additionally, consuming foods that are high in antioxidants and vitamins, such as blueberries and leafy greens, can help reduce inflammation and improve overall health.

It's also important to be mindful of portion sizes and avoid overeating, as well as to limit or avoid foods and drinks that can exacerbate stress, such as caffeine and alcohol. Taking the time to sit down and enjoy meals, free from distractions, can also have a positive impact on stress levels and provide a moment of relaxation in a busy day.

Incorporating healthy eating habits into your daily routine can be a simple yet effective way to manage stress. By nourishing your body with the right nutrients, you can support your physical and mental health and better handle the demands of daily life.

4.3: Exercise for Stress Relief

Exercise is a powerful tool for managing stress and improving overall health and well-being. Regular physical activity has been shown to reduce symptoms of anxiety and depression, boost mood and energy levels, and improve sleep quality. Additionally, exercise can help to reduce the levels of stress hormones in the body and improve the ability to cope with stressors.

One of the key benefits of exercise for stress management is that it provides an outlet for pent-up tension and frustration. Exercise can also serve as a form of meditation, helping to quiet the mind and bring a sense of calm and clarity. Whether it's through high-intensity interval training, yoga, or a simple walk in nature, physical activity can be a valuable tool for reducing stress and promoting mental and emotional well-being.

It's important to find an exercise routine that works best for you and your individual needs. Some people find that intense exercise provides the best stress relief, while others prefer more low-key activities like yoga or tai chi. Whatever your preference, the key is to find an activity that you enjoy and make it a regular part of your routine.

Incorporating exercise into your daily routine can have a profound impact on your stress levels and overall well-being. Whether it's through a structured workout program or simply taking the time to stretch and move your body, making physical activity a priority is a key component of a healthy and balanced life.

Chapter 4: Time Management and Prioritization

5.1 The Link between Time Management and Stress

In our fast-paced, modern world, stress is an inevitable part of life. It can come from a variety of sources, including work, family, and personal relationships. One common source of stress is poor time management. When we feel like we don't have enough time to get everything done, it can lead to feelings of overwhelm, frustration, and burnout.

However, time management is not just about having enough time to get things done. It's also about how we use that time and the impact it has on our stress levels. For example, when we procrastinate or waste time, it can increase our stress levels, as we feel like we're running out of time and can't keep up with our responsibilities. On the other hand, when we prioritize our time effectively, it can help us reduce stress, as we feel more in control and have a clearer understanding of what needs to be done.

In this chapter, we will explore the link between time management and stress, and how we can use time management strategies to reduce stress and improve our overall well-being. Whether you're a busy professional, a student, or a stay-at-home parent, you'll learn how to prioritize your time, manage your workload, and minimize stress in your daily life. With practical tips, techniques, and tools, you'll discover how to take control of your time and use it to achieve your goals and live a more fulfilling life.

Stress and time management are closely intertwined. Many of us experience stress due to feeling overwhelmed by the demands on our time and the constant pressure to balance work, personal life, and other responsibilities. When we struggle to manage our time effectively, we often feel rushed, frazzled, and stressed out, which can take a toll on our mental and physical health.

At the root of time management is the ability to prioritize and make intentional decisions about how we spend our time. When we feel in control of our schedule and have a clear understanding of what is most important, we can reduce the level of stress in our lives. On the other hand, when we don't have a handle on our schedule and feel like we're always playing catch-up, stress levels can skyrocket.

The good news is that time management skills can be learned and improved, and incorporating healthy habits like prioritization and planning can help us manage stress and lead a more fulfilling life.

5.2 Techniques for Effective Time Management

Time management and prioritization are two critical components in the pursuit of better mental health and overall well-being. In today's fast-paced and demanding world, it's easy to become overwhelmed and stressed, but with the right techniques and strategies, you can take control of your time and effectively manage your priorities.

Let us explore several techniques for effective time management and prioritization, including:

Creating a to-do list - This is one of the most straightforward and effective methods for managing your time and priorities. Write down all of the tasks you need to complete and prioritize them according to their importance and urgency. This helps you keep track of your progress and provides a sense of accomplishment as you cross off each item on your list.

Planning ahead - Take the time to plan out your day, week, or month ahead of time. This helps you to anticipate challenges and prioritize your tasks more effectively. By having a clear understanding of what you need to do, you can focus your energy and attention on the most important tasks, leading to greater productivity and less stress.

Making use of technology - There are numerous tools and apps available that can help you manage your time and priorities, from simple calendars to sophisticated project management software. Make use of these resources to stay organized, keep track of deadlines, and manage your tasks more effectively.

Taking breaks - Regular breaks are essential for maintaining your mental health and well-being. Take a few minutes to stretch, meditate, or simply relax, and you'll return to your work feeling refreshed and energized.

Learning to say no - One of the biggest challenges in time management and prioritization is learning to say no. It's important to recognize when you have too much on your plate and to prioritize your own well-being. Saying no to certain tasks or commitments can help you avoid burnout and maintain a better work-life balance.

By implementing these techniques, you can take control of your time, manage your priorities, and improve your mental health and overall well-being.

5.3 Setting Priorities and Boundaries

Setting priorities and boundaries is an essential component of effective time management and achieving better mental health and well-being. In today's demanding world, it can be easy to become overwhelmed and stressed, but with the right strategies and techniques, you can take control of your time and manage your priorities more effectively.

In this section, we will explore the importance of setting priorities and boundaries and the strategies you can use to achieve this.

Understanding your values - The first step in setting priorities and boundaries is to understand your values and what is most important to you. This can include your personal and professional goals, your relationships, and your health and well-being. By prioritizing these values, you can ensure that your time and energy are focused on the things that matter most to you.

Setting realistic goals - Once you understand your values, the next step is to set realistic goals. These goals should align with your values and be achievable within a specific time frame. By setting and working towards these goals, you can ensure that your time and energy are focused on what is most important to you.

Establishing boundaries - Boundaries are essential in maintaining a healthy work-life balance and avoiding burnout. This can include setting limits on the amount of time you spend working, the types of tasks you will and will not do, and the people you will and will not work with. By establishing these boundaries, you can ensure that your time and energy are focused on what is most important to you.

Prioritizing self-care - Self-care is an essential component of mental health and well-being, and it's important to prioritize this in your life. This can include activities such as exercise, meditation, and spending time with friends and family. By prioritizing self-care, you can ensure that you have the energy and focus to effectively manage your priorities.

Saying no - One of the most important aspects of setting priorities and boundaries is learning to say no. It's essential to recognize when you have too much on your plate and to prioritize your own well-being. Saying no to certain tasks or commitments can help you avoid burnout and maintain a better work-life balance.

Therefore, setting priorities and boundaries is an essential component of effective time management and achieving better mental health and well-being. By understanding your values, setting realistic goals, establishing boundaries, prioritizing self-care, and saying no when necessary, you can take control of your time and manage your priorities more effectively.

Chapter 5: Coping with Difficult Situations

6.1 Coping with Workplace Stress

Workplace stress is a common challenge for many individuals in today's fast-paced and demanding world. Stress in the workplace can impact your mental health, productivity, and overall well-being, but with the right strategies and techniques, you can learn to cope effectively.

In this section, we will explore strategies for coping with workplace stress, including:

Identifying stressors - The first step in coping with workplace stress is to identify the sources of stress. This can include factors such as heavy workloads, difficult colleagues, and tight deadlines. By recognizing these stressors, you can develop strategies to mitigate their impact on your mental health and well-being.

Practicing self-care - Self-care is an essential component of managing stress and maintaining your mental health and well-being. This can include activities such as exercise, meditation, and spending time with friends and family. By prioritizing self-care, you can ensure that you have the energy and focus to effectively manage stress in the workplace.

Seeking support - Don't be afraid to seek support from friends, family, or a mental health professional. Talking about your stressors can help you process your emotions and develop strategies for managing them more effectively.

Setting boundaries - It's important to set boundaries in the workplace to avoid burnout and maintain a healthy work-life balance. This can include setting limits on the amount of time you spend working, the types of tasks you will and will not do, and the people you will and will not work with. By establishing these boundaries, you can ensure that your time and energy are focused on what is most important to you.

Time management and prioritization - Effective time management and prioritization can help you manage your workload and reduce stress in the workplace. By prioritizing your tasks, delegating when necessary, and seeking help when you need it, you can ensure that your workload is manageable and your stress levels remain under control.

6.2 Dealing with Family and Relationship Stress

Family and relationship stress is a common challenge for many individuals, but with the right strategies and techniques, you can learn to cope effectively. Stress in your personal relationships can impact your mental health, productivity, and overall well-being, but with the right tools, you can manage this stress and maintain healthy, positive relationships.

In this section, we will explore strategies for coping with family and relationship stress, including:

Communicating effectively - Effective communication is key to managing stress in your personal relationships. By openly and honestly communicating your feelings, needs, and expectations, you can reduce misunderstandings and resolve conflicts more effectively.

Practicing self-care - Self-care is an essential component of managing stress and maintaining your mental health and well-being. This can include activities such as exercise, meditation, and spending time with friends and family. By prioritizing self-care, you can ensure that you have the energy and focus to effectively manage stress in your personal relationships.

Seeking support - Don't be afraid to seek support from friends, family, or a mental health professional. Talking about your stressors can help you process your emotions and develop strategies for managing them more effectively.

Setting boundaries - It's important to set boundaries in your personal relationships to avoid burnout and maintain a healthy work-life balance. This can include setting limits on the amount of time you spend with certain individuals, the types of tasks you will and will not do, and the types of interactions you will and will not engage in. By establishing these boundaries, you can ensure that your time and energy are focused on what is most important to you.

Making time for your relationships - Maintaining healthy, positive relationships requires time and effort, and it's important to prioritize this in your life. Whether it's spending quality time with your partner, friends, or family, making time for your relationships can help you manage stress and maintain your mental health and well-being.

6.3 Coping with Financial Stress

Financial stress is a common challenge for many individuals, but with the right strategies and techniques, you can learn to cope effectively. Stress related to finances can impact your mental health, productivity, and overall well-being, but with the right tools, you can manage this stress and regain control over your financial life.

In this section, we will explore strategies for coping with financial stress, including:

Creating a budget - The first step in coping with financial stress is to create a budget. By tracking your income and expenses, you can gain a clear understanding of your financial situation and develop a plan to manage your finances more effectively.

Reducing expenses - Reducing expenses is a key component of managing financial stress. This can include cutting back on unnecessary spending, negotiating bills and expenses, and finding ways to save money in your daily life.

Seeking professional help - If your financial situation is particularly challenging, don't hesitate to seek help from a financial advisor or credit counselor. These professionals can provide guidance and support to help you regain control over your finances and reduce stress.

Building an emergency fund - Building an emergency fund is an important step in managing financial stress. By setting aside money each month, you can ensure that you have the resources you need to cope with unexpected expenses and financial emergencies.

Staying informed - Staying informed about personal finance, budgeting, and financial planning is an important component of managing financial stress. Whether it's through reading books, attending workshops, or participating in online courses, staying informed can help you make better financial decisions and reduce stress.

It is evident that financial and relationship stress can greatly affect one's mental health and overall well-being. However, by adopting the right strategies and taking a proactive approach, you can effectively manage these types of stress and improve your quality of life.

Whether it's through creating a budget, communicating effectively, setting boundaries, or seeking professional help, you have the power to reduce stress and prioritize your mental health.

Remember, taking care of yourself should be a top priority, and by doing so, you can better handle the challenges of daily life and lead a more fulfilling life.

7.1 The Power of Positive Thinking.

Positive thinking has been shown to have numerous benefits for mental health and overall well-being. By focusing on the good and practicing gratitude, we can shift our perspective and create a more positive outlook on life.

Positive thinking can help us overcome challenges, reduce stress, and improve our relationships with others. When we adopt a positive outlook, we become more resilient and better equipped to handle difficult situations. We are also more likely to see opportunities, rather than obstacles, and to take action towards our goals.

One simple way to start incorporating positive thinking into your daily routine is by writing down three things you are grateful for each day. This practice can help shift your focus away from negative thoughts and towards the good in your life. Another technique is to reframe negative thoughts into positive ones. For example, instead of thinking "I can't do this," try thinking "I will find a way to do this."

The power of positive thinking is that it can become a self-fulfilling prophecy. When we focus on the positive, we become more confident, motivated, and optimistic. This, in turn, helps us to achieve our goals and create a more fulfilling life. So, take control of your thoughts and start thinking positively today! Your mental health and overall well-being will thank you for it.

7.2 Cultivating Gratitude and Optimism.

Gratitude and optimism are two essential components of a positive outlook on life. They are powerful tools that can help us to focus on the good, overcome challenges, and improve our mental health and well-being.

Gratitude involves taking the time to acknowledge and appreciate the good things in our lives. By focusing on what we have, rather than what we lack, we can cultivate a sense of contentment and joy. One way to practice gratitude is to write down three things you are grateful for each day. This simple act can help shift your focus away from negative thoughts and towards the positive.

Optimism, on the other hand, is a positive outlook on the future. It involves believing that things will work out for the best and that there is always a silver lining. Optimistic people are better equipped to handle challenges and setbacks because they see them as temporary setbacks, rather than permanent failures.

Together, gratitude and optimism can help us to cultivate a more positive outlook on life. By focusing on the good, we become more resilient and better equipped to handle difficult situations. We also become more motivated, confident, and optimistic, which helps us to achieve our goals and create a more fulfilling life. So, start practicing gratitude and cultivating optimism today! Your mental health and well-being will thank you for it.

7.3 Building a Support System.

Having a strong support system is crucial for maintaining a positive outlook on life. A support system provides us with a sense of connection, encouragement, and comfort, and helps us to handle life's challenges with grace and resilience.

Building a support system involves surrounding yourself with people who care about you, believe in you, and are there for you. This can include family, friends, colleagues, or even online communities. When you have a supportive network of people, you have someone to turn to when you need a listening ear, a shoulder to cry on, or a little extra encouragement.

It's important to nurture your relationships with the people in your support system. Take the time to invest in your relationships by showing appreciation, being there for others, and making time for them. This will help to build trust, deepen connections, and create a strong support network that you can rely on.

Having a support system can also help you to maintain a positive outlook by giving you a sense of purpose and belonging. When you know that you are valued and appreciated, you are more likely to feel confident, optimistic, and motivated. This can help you to handle life's challenges with greater resilience and overcome obstacles with a positive attitude.

Building a support system is an essential part of maintaining a positive outlook on life. By surrounding yourself with supportive people and investing in your relationships, you can create a network of support that will help you to handle life's challenges and maintain a positive outlook, no matter what comes your way. So, start building your support system today and watch your outlook on life transform for the better!

Chapter 7: Seeking Professional Help

8.1 When to Seek Help for Stress Management.

Managing stress is an important aspect of maintaining your mental health and well-being, and seeking professional help can be an effective way to achieve this. However, it's not always easy to know when it's time to seek help.

Here are some signs that indicate it may be time to seek help for stress management:

Persistent feelings of anxiety or depression: If you are experiencing persistent feelings of anxiety, depression, or both, it may be time to seek help. These feelings can impact your daily life and make it difficult to cope with stress.

Difficulty sleeping: Stress can interfere with your ability to get a good night's sleep. If you are having trouble sleeping, it may be time to seek help from a professional.

Substance abuse: If you have started to use drugs or alcohol to cope with stress, it's a clear sign that you need to seek help. Substance abuse can lead to a range of serious health problems and make it even harder to manage stress.

Physical symptoms: Chronic stress can lead to physical symptoms such as headaches, muscle tension, and digestive problems. If you are experiencing physical symptoms that you believe are related to stress, it's a good idea to seek help.

Difficulty managing daily tasks: If stress is making it difficult for you to complete daily tasks, it may be time to seek help. Professional support can help you to develop effective coping strategies that will make it easier for you to manage stress and get back on track.

Seeking professional help for stress management is a vital aspect of maintaining your mental health and well-being. If you are experiencing persistent feelings of anxiety or depression, difficulty sleeping, substance abuse, physical symptoms, or difficulty managing daily tasks, it may be time to seek help. By seeking support from a professional, you can learn effective strategies for managing stress, reduce its impact on your life, and improve your overall sense of well-being.

8.2 Types of Professional Help for Stress Management

When it comes to managing stress, it's important to understand that everyone's needs are different. As such, there are a number of different types of professional help available to help you manage stress and improve your mental health. Here are some of the most common types of professional help for stress management:

Therapy or Counseling: Talking to a mental health professional, such as a therapist or counselor, can be an effective way to manage stress and improve your mental health. Through therapy, you can work through difficult emotions and experiences, develop coping strategies, and build resilience against stress.

Medication: In some cases, medication can be an effective way to manage stress and improve your mental health. Antidepressants, for example, can help manage depression and anxiety, which are common sources of stress.

Complementary and Alternative Medicine (CAM): CAM treatments, such as acupuncture, massage therapy, and mindfulness practices, can be used to complement traditional medical treatment and help manage stress.

Lifestyle Changes: Making changes to your lifestyle, such as exercise, healthy eating, and sleep, can help improve your overall health and reduce stress. Your doctor or mental health professional can provide guidance on how to make these changes effectively.

It's important to note that professional help should be sought out when you are feeling overwhelmed and unable to manage stress on your own. If you are feeling hopeless, having thoughts of suicide, or experiencing other symptoms of a mental health condition, it's important to seek help immediately.

8.3: The Benefits of Therapy for Stress Management

As individuals, we all face stress and challenges in our daily lives. It is a normal part of the human experience, and at times, stress can even be motivating and drive us to succeed. However, when stress becomes persistent and overwhelming, it can start to take a toll on our mental and physical health. This is when seeking professional help can be beneficial.

One of the most effective ways to manage stress is through therapy. Therapy is a process in which individuals work with a trained professional to identify the sources of their stress and develop coping strategies to manage it. Therapy can be conducted one-on-one, in a group setting, or even online.

There are many benefits to seeking therapy for stress management. Some of these benefits include:

Improved coping skills: A trained therapist can help individuals identify the sources of their stress and develop coping skills to manage it. They can also teach individuals how to identify when stress is becoming overwhelming and provide strategies to manage it in a healthy and effective way.

Increased self-awareness: Therapy can help individuals gain insight into their thoughts, emotions, and behaviors. This increased self-awareness can be helpful in understanding the sources of stress and developing effective coping strategies.

Improved mental health: Therapy can help individuals with depression, anxiety, and other mental health issues that can contribute to stress. By working through these issues, individuals can improve their overall mental health and reduce stress.

Better relationships: Therapy can help individuals improve their relationships with others. By working through communication and relationship issues, individuals can reduce stress and improve their overall quality of life.

Better physical health: Chronic stress has been linked to numerous physical health problems, including high blood pressure, heart disease, and stroke. By managing stress through therapy, individuals can reduce the risk of these health problems and improve their overall physical health.

Seeking help through therapy is a valuable investment in one's mental and physical health. A trained therapist can provide individuals with the tools they need to manage stress effectively and improve their overall well-being. So, if you're feeling overwhelmed by stress, consider reaching out to a therapist today. Your future self will thank you.

Conclusion:

9.1 Summary of Key Points

In this modern world, stress has become a ubiquitous part of our daily lives. It is important to understand that while stress is a normal part of life, it can become overwhelming and start to negatively impact our mental and physical health. This guide has aimed to provide individuals with the tools and information they need to manage stress effectively in the 21st century.

Throughout this guide, we have discussed various strategies for managing stress, including:

Mindfulness and meditation: Practicing mindfulness and meditation can help individuals manage stress by reducing feelings of anxiety and improving their overall well-being.

Exercise and physical activity: Regular exercise has been shown to reduce stress and improve overall mental health.

Good sleep hygiene: Getting adequate sleep is essential for managing stress and improving overall mental health.

Healthy diet: Eating a well-balanced diet that includes plenty of fruits, vegetables, and whole grains can help reduce stress and improve overall physical health.

Seeking professional help: If stress becomes persistent and overwhelming, seeking professional help through therapy can be beneficial.

9.2 The Importance of Continual Stress Management

Managing stress is a continuous process and requires continual effort. The strategies outlined in this guide can help individuals reduce stress and improve their mental health, but it's important to remember that stress is a normal part of life and can resurface at any time. This is why it's essential to continually implement stress management techniques in one's daily life.

Incorporating stress management techniques into your daily routine can help reduce the negative impact of stress and improve your overall well-being. This can include practising mindfulness and meditation, engaging in regular physical activity, maintaining good sleep hygiene, and eating a well-balanced diet. It's also important to seek professional help if stress becomes persistent and overwhelming.

Additionally, it's important to identify your personal stress triggers and develop effective coping strategies. This may involve learning new relaxation techniques, practicing self-care, or seeking support from friends, family, or a therapist. It's also important to prioritize your mental health and make time for activities that bring you joy and relaxation.

9.3 Final Thoughts on Living a Stress-Free Life

Living a stress-free life may seem like an impossible dream, but with the right tools and techniques, it can become a reality. By implementing the strategies discussed in this guide, individuals can reduce the negative impact of stress and improve their overall well-being.

It's important to remember that everyone experiences stress differently, and what works for one person may not work for another. However, by incorporating a multi-faceted approach to stress management, individuals can find what works best for them. This may involve a combination of mindfulness and meditation, exercise and physical activity, good sleep hygiene, a healthy diet, and seeking professional help if needed.

It is very important to prioritize self-care and make time for activities that bring joy and relaxation. This can include spending time with loved ones, engaging in hobbies, or simply taking a break from the demands of daily life.

In summary, mastering your mental health in the 21st century requires a multi-faceted approach that includes mindfulness and meditation, exercise, good sleep hygiene, a healthy diet, self-care, and seeking professional help if needed. This approach can help reduce the negative impact of stress and improve overall well-being. Taking care of your mental health is just as important as taking care of your physical health and requires effort and dedication. By prioritizing self-care and implementing stress management techniques into your daily routine, you can achieve a stress-less life. Remember, investing in yourself is the best investment you can make, so take control of your mental health today and start

living a stress-free life.

<u>**Appendix: Additional Resources for Stress Management**</u>

In this appendix, we will provide a list of additional resources for those looking to further explore and deepen their knowledge of stress management. These resources include books, websites, and support groups that offer practical advice, tips, and techniques for managing stress and improving mental health.

Books:

"The Stress-Proof Brain: Master Your Emotional Response to Stress Using Mindfulness and Neuroplasticity" by Melanie Greenberg

"The Anxiety Survival Guide for Teens: CBT Skills to Overcome Fear, Worry, and Panic" by Jennifer Shannon

"The Power of Now: A Guide to Spiritual Enlightenment" by Eckhart Tolle

"Mindfulness: An Eight-Week Plan for Finding Peace in a Frantic World" by Mark Williams and Danny Penman

Websites:

Headspace (www.headspace.com)

Calm (www.calm.com)

Mindful (www.mindful.org)

Anxiety and Depression Association of America (www.adaa.org)

Support Groups:

National Alliance on Mental Illness (www.nami.org)

Anxiety and Depression Support Group (www.anxietydepressionsupportgroup.org)

Depression and Bipolar Support Alliance (www.dbsalliance.org)

Local Support Groups and Workshops

In addition to online resources, there are also local support groups and workshops available for those seeking help with stress management. These groups provide a supportive community of individuals who are going through similar experiences and offer a safe space to share and discuss coping strategies. Some popular organizations that offer local support groups and workshops include:

National Alliance on Mental Illness (NAMI)

Anxiety and Depression Association of America (ADAA)

Depression and Bipolar Support Alliance (DBSA)

Mental Health America

These organizations offer a range of services, including support groups, educational workshops, and advocacy and awareness events. Attending these events can help provide practical skills and techniques for managing stress, as well as the opportunity to connect with others who are going through similar experiences.